The Big Book Of Essential Oil Recipes For Healing & Health

Over 200 Aromatherapy Remedies For Common Ailments

MEL HAWLEY

ISBN-13:978-1535035620

ISBN-10:1535035625

DEDICATION

All things bright and beautiful

All creatures great and small

All things wise and wonderful

The Lord God made them all

TABLE OF CONTENTS

INTRODUCTION

Essential Oils, Healing & Aromatherapy

Essential oils are highly concentrated substances extracted from the leaves, bark, bushes, flowers, roots, fruits, shrubs or seeds of plants. They are beautifully and uniquely fragrant and give plants their distinctive smells. They also enhance plants' immune system and offer them the necessary protection. Each essential oil comes with its own individual scent, color, chemical properties and healing benefits. Additionally, essential oils evaporate easily into the air, absorb effortlessly into the skin when applied and never go rancid.

Essential oil is extracted from plants via many ways but the most common of them is steam distillation, a process which separates the oil and water-based plant compounds. The plants they are extracted from contain very powerful healing compounds. This is why they (essential oil) retain the very powerful healing properties of their mother plant.

Additionally, Essential oils are highly concentrated with a strong aroma. At times, it takes just one drop to provide the much needed great health benefits. However, that one drop may be extracted from a large quantity of plants. For instance, one pound of lavender essential oil is extracted from about 150 pounds of lavender flowers! Do you see how highly concentrated

1

essential oils are? So essentially (no pun meant), you will be getting 150 times the healing properties from lavender essential oils than you would get from using straight lavender flower.

While it is beneficial to utilize the health benefits of certain plants, such as ground ginger root and cinnamon for healing; and to eat healthy foods like fresh herbs and vegetables to maintain optimum health; essential oils, with its highly concentrated healing properties, remains the most potent form of plant based medicine, surpassing even dried herbs and medicinal tincture.

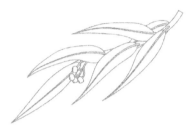

Essential oils have been in use for thousands of years to heal and purify the body of ailments and diseases. The ancient people discovered that the aromatic compounds in essential oils have direct effect on their mental, emotional and physical health. This is aromatherapy: the art of treating diseases with herbal essences. So effective is essential oil's power to heal and cure diseases, that a lot of people can now successfully avoid taking a plethora of medications or undergoing various surgeries, simply by taking essential oils correctly.

Essential oils are an amazing alternative medical treatment. However, they are complimentary and must never be regarded as a substitute to professional medical care. Aromatherapy alone (the use of essential oils for treatments) cannot cure a major illness or permanently cure your stress. What they do is to help in alleviating the symptoms of a physical condition and to temporarily eliminate stress or other psychological factors.

Also important, essential oil must be diluted with a carrier oil such as coconut or olive oil before they can be used. Once these oil compounds are in your system, they travel at an incredibly rate to protect and heal your body in a variety of ways.

Some Essential Oils And Their Functions

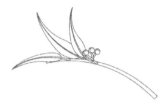

There are more than 100 different types of essential oils in the market. Amazingly, each of these oils contains its own special scent and properties that are applicable to many different conditions. Here are some popular essential oils and their uses:

- Eucalyptus: invigorating and purifying, it is often used in topical preparations but do not apply to children's face.
- Ginger: helps to stimulate the appetite and relieves headaches.
- Lavender: promotes a relaxed and calm feeling.
- Lemon: joyful oil that also refreshes but should be diluted well if applying to the skin.
- Peppermint: filled with powerfully minty aroma, peppermint oil is refreshing and cooling.
- Rosemary: This clarifying fragrance is generally used in shampoos, household sprays and soaps.

- <u>Sage</u>: has a warming camphor scent and you need just one drop to experience it.
- <u>Tea Tree:</u> helps to fight against bacteria, viruses and fungi and stimulate the body's immune system.
- <u>Ylang Ylang</u>: originally cultivated in the Philippines, the ylang ylang plant soon became widespread due to its distinctive scent and look. This essential oil helps to relax the mind and body.
- <u>Clove</u> a versatile oil, it provides relief from aches and pains such as headache, tooth and gum pain, earache and stomach ache. It is also useful for skin ailments such as bug bites and cuts.

Kid- friendly essential oils include lavender, lemon, grapefruit, pine, tea tree, spruce and peppermint for kids above 6 years of age.

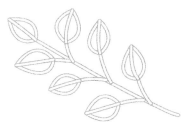

Is This Essential Oil Good For Me?

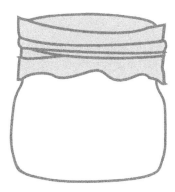

Not everyone responds to essential oil treatment in the same way. This is because essential oils comprise different characteristics so they should be handled differently. 'Stronger or hotter' oils for instance can cause skin irritation for many people. An essential oil that doesn't irritate you can still irritate someone else. Also, if you are allergic to a specific plant, there is a tendency for you to also be allergic to the essential oil where it is extracted from.

For this reason, it is advisable to do a skin patch test to verify its safeness on your skin.

How to Perform a Skin Patch Test

• Combine 1 drop of essential oil and half a teaspoon of carrier oil (olive or jojoba oil will do). Place 1-2 drops of this combination on the inside of your elbow, wrist or underside of the forearm.

• You may apply a bandage to avoid getting the area wet.

• If you feel any irritation, itching or notice some redness, take away the bandage immediately and wash the area carefully.

• If no irritation happens after a few hours, you can go ahead and use the essential oil in diluted form as it is safe on your skin.

Ascertaining Quality

The quality of essential oils matter a lot. Not all essential oils are created the same. When purchasing essential oils, make sure they are pure and of high quality. Do not buy fragrance oils or diluted essentials oils. The therapeutic properties are in the actual substances and not just the fragrance.

Cheap copies bring cheap results, causing problems like skin irritation or even worsening an already existing ailment. There is no regulating body for essential oils so you need to buy from trusted and reputable source to enjoy effective results. Be wary of mislabeled products. Just because a labeled bottle indicates quality doesn't necessarily mean the content can be trusted.

To test if your oils are pure, put 3-4 drops on a blotting paper. Pure essential oil will evaporate quickly leaving no trace but petroleum solvents and adulterated essential oils will. The presence of a noticeable ring indicates that the oil is diluted.

There Are Four Grades Of Essential Oils:

1. Synthetic and Altered Oils are the lowest grade of oil. They are created in laboratory.

2. Natural and "Pure" Oils. They are the most commonly sold type of oils. They are usually over-processed so they lose their healing compounds.

3. Wellness Grade Essential Oils; these are steam distilled with healing compounds. The only setback is that they may have been sprayed with pesticides.

4. Certified Therapeutic Grade Essential Oils; these are the highest grade of essential oils with maximum healing properties.

Finally, bottle the oils in dark glass containers to protect from sunlight and oxidation. Ensure you buy therapeutic grade and organic oils at all times when purchasing essential oils.

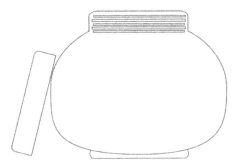

Diluting Essential Oils With Carrier Oils

Carrier oils are pressed from the fatty portions of plants such as the seeds and nuts. As a result, most of them have minimal aroma and minimal color. Some of them also last for a short while as they become rancid after a while. Carrier oils also act as a lubricating agent during massage of larger areas and muscles. They aid absorption as well. Unlike essential oils that evaporate easily when diluted, carrier oils do not.

Ideal carrier oils for essential oils include olive oil, jojoba, sweet almond oil, pomegranate seed oil, pecan oil, evening primrose oil, hemp seed oil, sesame oil, avocado oil, rose hip oil, sunflower oil and many more.

In order to retain the freshness of your carrier oils, keep them from direct light and heat. Make small batches of blends that can be used within a short time. Jojoba oil is very helpful in extending the shelf life of your blend. Essential and carrier oils can also be refrigerated to extend their shelf life.

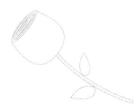

 A 2% dilution is ideal for most aromatherapy applications. Going beyond this measurement may lead to adverse effect. For children and the elderly and in dividuals with health issues, just 1% dilution of carrier oil is sufficient

Application And Dosage

Use essential oils sparingly and do not exceed the recommended dosage as they are very potent. As little as 1 to 2 drops will go a long way towards offering the therapeutic benefits that is required

The most effective and safest area of the body for applying essential oils is the bottom of the feet. This is very helpful for young children or people with frail health. The sole of our feet are thick and are unlikely to cause skin irritations. Thus, the feet are really great place to apply "hotter" oils and anti-infectious blends.

Also, there are lots of nerve endings on the soles of the feet which help to carry the oils quickly into the bloodstream. For example, if you rub a clove of garlic clove on the bottom of your foot, your breath will smell of garlic within 15 minutes!

To treat a particular area like a rash, burn, wound or sore muscle, apply the oils on the problem spot directly. Other safe areas for applying oils are the inside elbows and knees, the nape of the neck and base of the throat.

Another good area for applying essential oils is the scalp because the size of the hair follicle is much bigger than the skin pores. Essential oils penetrate the scalp easily when it is applied on it, stimulating it.

Essential oils can last between 12 - 24 hours in the body. However, certain factors such as the body area where the oils were applied, the application method (topical or inhalation), viscosity and skin type can diminish or extend the therapeutic duration.

Using Essential Oils

There are 3 main ways essential oils can be used: topical, inhalation and internal.

Topical Use

This involves applying essential oils on the skin, either directly or directly. A few oils can be applied directly on the skin e.g. lavender but most oils must be mixed with a carrier oil before usage. Some of the best carrier oils include jojoba oil, coconut oil, olive oil, almond oil and pomegranate seed oil.

Key points of application on the body are:

• Behind ears

• Abdomen

• Neck

• Temples

• Soles and tops of feet

• Along spine

• Upper back

Other Topical Ways To Use Oils Include:

Baths: essential oils can be used as aromatherapy baths.. This could help improve circulation, relax the body, relieve sore muscles, open airways, improve sleep and soothe the skin. It is best to mix the oils with bath salts, milk or sesame oil for quick dispersion. Failure to do this will cause the oils to float on water and even stick to your skin directly. Use soothing oils like lavender and eucalyptus. Additionally, the bath could either be a full body bath or foot bath.

Massage: Aromatherapy massage is another effective topical application. Make sure that you always dilute with suitable carrier oil.

Compresses: compresses work well for infections, bruises, aches and pains. Simply add your preferred essential oil to bowl of either hot or cold water. (It could be diluted with carrier, depending on the treatment). Dip a clean cloth in the water, wring it out and place on the affected area. Peppermint works real well for muscle aches and lavender is just great for infections.

Salves: to make salves, mix coconut oil, vitamin E oil, beeswax and essential oils. Store in a metal or glass container and rub as needed. Salves are very effective for cuts, scrapes, bruises or sore muscle.

Inhalation

Diffusion is another excellent way to use essential oil. You can either use diffusers or inhale the oil directly in hot water. Inhalations are highly effective for headaches, respiratory and sinus problems. Only ensure that you inhale for 2- 3 minutes at a stretch. Inhaling essential oils for too long can cause nausea, dizziness and headaches.

Internal Use

Internal use of essential oils can only be effective if pure therapeutic grade oils are used. Dosage and dilution is also dependent on the individual's age, size and health. However, it is best to consult your physician or nutritionist before ingesting any essential oil.

Ways by which essential oils can be taken internally include:

• Putting a few drops in an empty capsule and swallowing with water

• Putting 1-3 drops of oil to 1 teaspoon of coconut oil then consume.

• Adding 1-3 drops of oil to a glass of coconut milk, water or almond milk.

• Adding 1-3 drops of oil to 1 teaspoon of raw honey.

Others are:

Insect Repellent

Many essential oils such as peppermint, lavender and citronella act as a natural repellent against insects. To repel insects, sprinkle some drops of essential oil onto tissues or cotton balls and place them near your doors and windows. Make sure you go through the safety information on the oils you intend to use because some oils may be unsuitable for usage around pets. Also, do not apply the oil directly on fragile surfaces.

Basic Precautions For Essential Oils Usage

- <u>Pregnancy</u>: Studies have shown that applying essential oils topically, and after the first trimester, cannot harm a developing fetus. Nevertheless, it is still advisable to consult a seasoned aromatherapist before usage.

- <u>Eyes And Ears</u>: Be careful with sensitive parts of the body like the eyes and ears. Never apply essential oils directly to the ear canal or the eyes. Wash your hand thoroughly after application in order to avoid actions like rubbing the eyes, touching the interior of the nose or handling contact lenses.

- <u>Babies and Those with Sensitive Skin:</u> Take extra care with babies and individuals with sensitive skin. Extra caution should be taken when treating babies, small children, and the elderly. This is because they have very sensitive skin that is prone to burning, irritation or stinging sensations. Protect the skin against irritation by using an effective base or carrier oil.

- <u>Natural Elements</u>: Some essential oils, mostly citrus oils react to radiant energy, light or other sources of UV rays. Once applied, a rash on the skin or a dark pigmentation shows up within hours or days. It is best to wait for about 6 hours after using any of these photosensitizing oils before exposing the skin to sunlight.

- <u>Keep Out of Reach of Children</u>: Just as you would for medicine, treat essential oils the same way. Essential oils wrongly ingested are just as harmful and painful as if accidentally used in the eyes. Do not be carried away with the fragrances emitting from these oils to forget that they can be hazardous in young children's hands.

- <u>Suspicious Claims</u>: Exercise caution with companies that state their product as "Made With Natural Ingredients" or "Made With Essential Oils". Claims like this do not explicitly state that the product is only made with the specified ingredient. It is possible for such products to contain a tiny amount of essential oil just so that they can make the "Made with Essential Oils" claim.

- <u>The Lesser The Better</u>: Always remember that these oils are highly concentrated so be sure to follow the exact usage. If one drop can deliver the expected results, do not use two.

Others include:

- Do not use undiluted essential oils on your skin. With the exception of lavender and tea tree oils (Melaleuca), on no account should you use any essential oil in its pure form.
- Individuals with health conditions like epilepsy and asthma must seek a doctor's approval.
- Not all essential oils can be used in aromatherapy. Pennyroyal, Wormood, Camphor, Onion, Sassafras, Horseradish, Bitter Almond and Rue are some of these essential oils.
- Do not use essential oils on damaged or chemically- burned skin.
- Wash hands thoroughly after application so you do not leave essential oil residue on your fingers. This may damage contact lenses and cause eye discomfort.
- Wear disposable latex gloves when working with essential oils as this will prevent inflammation or itchy skin.
- Always work in an area with good ventilation.
- Most essential oils are flammable so keep them from open flame or spark.

Top Essential Oils For Healing

Stock these essential oils in your medicine cabinet and keep your family healthy all year long.

<u>Lemon</u>

Lemon oil is effective in its ability to detox every part of the body. With its uplifting properties, it is also good for improved focus, concentration and to rejuvenate energy. It helps treat wounds and infections and acts as a powerful bug repellent.

<u>Uses</u>

• To freshen breath, put 1-2 drops in water.

• To promote cleansing & metabolism, take 1 drop as supplement three times daily.

• To uplift mood, diffuse to clean air and enjoy a nice citrus scent.

• Improve home smell by diffusing in the air.

• Rub on hands in instead of hand sanitizer for its antimicrobial benefits.

• Mix with baking soda as all- natural teeth whitener.

• Mix with olive oil and use as natural cleaning product.

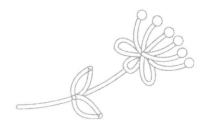

Lavender

One of the most versatile oils, lavender has antiviral and antibacterial properties and it is effective on cuts, bruises and general skin care. It doesn't always require a carrier oil and can be applied directly to the affected area. It is relaxing and uplifting, helping to balance hormones in women and generally reducing the stress hormones in the body.

Uses

• To relax the body and improve sleep, rub on neck in the evenings.

• To restore the body after a long day, add a few drops to your bath along with some Epsom salts.

• Put on your kids' cuts, bruises, scrapes, burns, rashes, and wounds.

• Diffuse in the air improve mood and relax.

• Use topically on neck to lower cholesterol& blood pressure or take as supplement.

Tea Tree

Also called Melaleuca, tea tree is a powerful antifungal, antibacterial and antiseptic oil. It can be used topically to treat all sorts of skin problems. You only need a few drops diluted with a carrier oil and your cuts, scrapes, acne blemishes, insect bites, ringworm, warts, fungal infections, athletic foot and even dandruff will be eliminated. It can also help to boost the immune system. In some cases, it can even be used undiluted. It is found in a lot of skin care products.

Uses

• Mix 5 drops with 1 tablespoon of raw honey and use mixture as acne free -face wash.

• Apply to ringworm, Candida, athlete's foot or other fungal infections.

• Put directly on mosquito, spider or bug bites to detox poison.

• Add 5 drops to your favorite shampoo to reduce dandruff and to improve scalp health.

• Kick a cold or flu by gargling tea tree oil and water.

• Mix 2 teaspoon of melaleuca and water in a spray bottle for an all-purpose cleaner.

• Diffuse in the air to purify it of mold and allergens.

Peppermint:

Peppermint is cooling, it stimulates the mind and increases mental alertness. For an instant cooling effect, simply dilute with a carrier and rub on your chest, back and neck. Peppermint oil wards off nausea, morning or motion sickness.

 It reduces headaches and migraines to a large extent when applied to the temple. It has antimicrobial properties as well so also helps to freshen bad breath and treat digestive issues such as flatulence, indigestion and slow digestion.

Uses

• Mix with coconut oil or carrier oil of choice and rub topically on sore muscles.

• Diffuse it in air to improve energy and focus.

• To improve breathing and fight infections, rub on bottom of feet& chest

• Mix with baking soda and coconut oil for homemade toothpaste.

• Freshen breath, put 1 drop in clean water.

•To improve digestion & reduce nausea, take 1 drop in water.

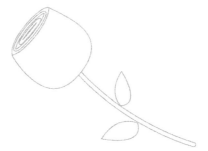

Frankincense

A very powerful essential oil, frankincense was valued above gold in ancient times due its ability to treat all sorts of illnesses. Recent research has shown that it is even more effective than chemotherapy in shrinking tumors and killing cancer cells. It helps to reduce inflammation and improve immune function. It also fights infections, heals acne, sunspot and skin scarring.

Uses

• To improve immunity, rub topically on neck, chest, behind ears and to bottoms of feet.

• Apply to minor cuts for healing and pain relief.

• To reduce scars, age spots and stretch marks, dilute oil and apply once or twice a day.

• Use after a trauma to calm yourself.

• Rub topically on areas of joint pain

• To relieve stress and headaches, apply to temples with lavender.

• Add to baths for extra relaxation.

• Diffuse in air to reduce seasonal allergies

Eucalyptus

This is a powerful antiviral, antibacterial and antispasmodic oil that works on coughs, colds and allergies that affect breathing. To clear your nasal passages and lungs, just add a few drops to a vaporizer or to bowl of steaming water and inhale. It stimulates the immune system and loosens congested chest. Prevent a full cold also by using regularly during cold season.

Sandalwood

A powerful fighter of bacteria and viruses, sandalwood essential oil, offers a host of benefits to the skin when properly applied. Let's consider a few of these applications.

To fight rashes, itchiness or inflammation, combine 3-7 drops of sandalwood, one teaspoon of lime juice and one teaspoon of turmeric powder. Apply thinly to the skin and leave for 20- 30 minutes. Rinse with cool water and pat gently to dry. Redness or swelling may take time to subside but itchiness should quickly fade.

Sandalwood helps to even skin tone so if you have uneven tans, mix 7-10 drops of sandalwood with five teaspoons of coconut oil and two teaspoons of jojoba oil. Massage this blend into overexposed areas.

For pimples and acne, combine 3 to 7 drops of sandalwood essential oil, one teaspoon of spring water or rosewater and one teaspoon of turmeric powder. Apply thinly to the skin and leave for about thirty minutes. Rinse face with lukewarm water and gently dry. Do this one or two times daily and noticeable changes will be observed after only 48 hours.

An excellent moisturizer, sandalwood can aid dry skin. For specific areas, just apply 1-2 diluted drops to skin and massage. For a full body application, dilute with a carrier oil like jojoba oil and your skin will feel soft and hydrated.

To treat bug bite, mix 5 to 7 drops of sandalwood with one teaspoon of lavender oil, one teaspoon of turmeric and just enough water for a paste. Apply this paste to the bug bite immediately to reduce swelling and stop itching.

In addition, sandalwood oil is helpful for respiratory problems via steam inhalation. It is also great for conditioning dry hair. Simply apply 4-6 drops of it to your hair after a shower and your hair will be moisturized, soft and shiny.

COLDS AND FLUS

A cold is a viral infection of the nose and throat. Its symptoms include a sore throat, stuffed-up, runny nose, dry cough and sneezing.

Flu viruses are more infectious, more harmful and often stronger than those of colds. As a matter of fact, flu is a severe form of cold. It causes body aches, high fever, chills, exhaustion and muscle sores. Flu is highly contagious as well.

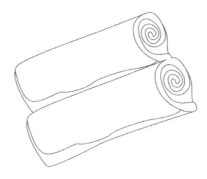

Anti-Flu Bath

4 drops Tea tree oil

3 drops Lavender oil

1 drop of Lemon oil

Instructions

Add all the essential oils to a warm bath.

Anti- Flu Massage

3 drops Tea tree oil

2 drops Eucalyptus oil

10 ml Evening primrose oil

Instructions

Add together and massage entire body after using the anti-flu bath oil.

Cream Recipe For Cold

2 drops of rosemary

2 drops of lavender

2 drops of eucalyptus

2 teaspoons of milk or cream

Instructions

1. Add the essential oils to cream or milk.

2. Make a warm bath, pour oils into it and enjoy.

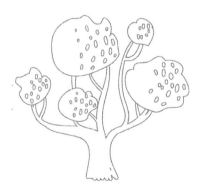

Feet Remedy For Cold & Chilly Feelings

6 drops of Geranium essential oil

10 drops of Lemon essential oil

4 drops of Rosemary essential oil

Instructions

1. Blend all together in an amber bottle.

2. In a large basin of not too hot water, add 3-4 drops.

3. Soak feet for 30 minutes or less.

4. Once done, dry your feet thoroughly and then apply a little lotion.

5. Put on your socks, slippers or shoes.

Colds & Flu Homemade Spray

1 drop of Niaouli essential oil

1 drop of Pine essential oil

1 drop of Cinnamon essential oil

1 drop of Cloves essential oil

1 drop of Eucalyptus essential oil

500 ml water

Instructions

1. Add the oils to the water, shake to combine and put in a spray can.

2. Spray the home.

Night-Time Colds & Flu Combater

2 drops Lavender

2 drops Tea Tree

What To Do

1. Add oils to a steaming bowl of water.

2. Let the steam diffuse into the room.

3. Alternatively, add oils to a tea candle diffuser.

RESPIRATORY TROUBLES

Breathing Rub For Asthma

The best time to treat asthma is in-between attacks. The wheezing sounds that asthma sufferers produce occur when air is released through the swollen and narrowed bronchial passages. To avoid adverse reaction, however, do a sniff test before using this recipe.

1 oz of Jojoba oil

2 drops of Frankincense essential oil

2 drops of Thyme essential oil

2 drops of Myrrh essential oil

3 drops of Pine needle essential oil

3 drops of Eucalyptus essential oil

3 drops of Tea Tree essential oil

Instructions

1. Combine all the oils in a clean PET plastic bottle, shaking well.

2. Rub on the chest and the mid back as needed.

Anti-Asthma Steam

1/4 teaspoon of Eucalyptus essential oil

3 cups of Boiled water

Instructions

1. Add essential oils to boiled water.

2. Next, drape a towel over the back of the head and place face over steam. Breathe in the steam, taking breaks as needed.

3. Do 3 to 4 rounds of steam inhalation every day.

Bronchitis Relief

Bronchitis occurs when the passage ways in the lungs becomes congested and inflamed, causing breathing difficulty.

1 ounce of Sunflower oil

12 drops of Eucalyptus essential oil

5 drops of Peppermint essential oil

5 drops of Thyme essential oil

Instructions

1. Add all the ingredients together

2. Rub mixture gently on your throat and chest about 4-5 times a day.

Massage Oil For Sinusitis

Sinusitis is caused by allergies, tonsillitis, poor mouth hygiene, colds or the flu. The protective mucous membranes that is in your sinus cavities become compromised by germs or other irritants, leading to inflammation and infection. The symptoms include nosebleed, nasal congestion, ear pain, fatigue, headache, mild fever, pain around the eyes and cough.

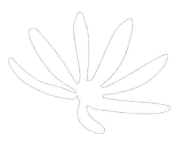

3 drops Geranium oil

2 drops Eucalyptus oil

2 drops Peppermint oil

3 drops Rosemary oil

1 drop Tea tree oil

10 ml carrier oil

Instructions

1. Add essential oils to any carrier oil of choice.

2. Massage the neck, nose, around the nose, forehead, and cheekbones. Also massage in front and behind the ears.

Essential Oil Therapy For Sinusitis

2 drops Tea tree essential oil

2 drops of Eucalyptus essential oil

1 drop of Thyme essential oil

1 drop of Ginger essential oil

2 quart of hot or steaming water

Instructions

1. Add the essential oils into the water.

2. Drape a towel over your head and then bend the head over the bowl. The towel should be draped over the bowl as well.

3. Breathe for 5 -10 minutes. Repeat this every day up to 6 times.

Sinusitis Steam Inhalation

2 drops Peppermint oil

1 drop Eucalyptus oil

2 drops Rosemary oil

Instructions

Use steam inhalation with these oils.

Hay Fever And Other Seasonal Allergies

Hay fever is an allergic reaction to pollen or dust. They occur quite spontaneously and usually affect the eyes and the upper respiratory tract. The symptoms include itching eyes, watering eyes, sneezing and runny nose.

3 drops Anise essential oil

3 drops Lemon essential oil

4 drops Eucalyptus essential oil

4 drops Chamomile essential oil

1 drops Petitgrain essential oil

5 ml Carrier oil of choice

Instructions

1. Properly blend oils in a dark bottle.

2. Use 15 to 20 drops in a bath

Hay Fever Care

Instructions

1. Put 2-3 drops of Eucalyptus, Tea Tree or Niaouli oil on a handkerchief.

2. Inhale whenever an attack occurs.

2. Alternatively, make a spray to spray in the room using diluted Eucalyptus oil

Vapor Rub For Chest Congestion

5 drops of Thyme essential oil

12 drops of Eucalyptus essential oil

5 drops of Peppermint essential oil

1 ounce of olive oil

Instructions

1. Combine all the ingredients in a glass bottle.

2. Shake very well to mix evenly.

3. Massage into chest and throat very gently.

4. Use 1-5 times daily and just before bed.

Nasal Inhaler For Chest Congestion

5 drops Eucalyptus essential oil

1/4 teaspoon coarse salt

Instructions

1. Place salt in a small glass bottle with a tight lid then add essential oil. (The work of the salt is to absorb the oil and keep it from spilling when it is carried).

2. When needed, open the vial and inhale deeply.

SORE THROAT, COUGH& CATARRH

Sore Throat Neck Wrap Treatment

Sore throat may be caused by bacterial infection, yelling, lots of talking or singing. Sometimes, the throat may be so inflamed that swallowing will be difficult.

2 drops Lavender essential oil

2 drops Bergamot essential oil

2 drops Tea tree essential oil

2 cups Hot water

Instructions

1. Mix essential oils with water. Soak a flannel in the still warm water, wring it out.

2. Wrap around neck and then cover with a thin towel to retain the heat. Take it off before it becomes cold. Use all through the day as frequently as you desire.

Throat Gargle &Spray For Sore Throat

4 drops Marjoram essential oil

1/2 cup Warm water

1/2 teaspoon Salt

Instructions

1. Add together all the ingredients.

2. Disperse the oils by shaking thoroughly and dissolve the salt before spraying or gargling.

 3. Gargle every 30 minutes first and then several times daily.

EO Gargle Method For Cough

Coughs have distinctive characteristics that can be recognized as either good or bad. The originating cause of a "bad" cough may be bacterial, viral or symptomatic of an entire different issue.

1- 2 drops of Peppermint, Eucalyptus, Lemon or essential oil

Instructions

1. Put oil(s) in a mouthful (about an ounce) of water.

2. Gargle and swallow if you want.

Rectifying Wet Throat Cough

2 drops Peppermint essential oil

2 drops Rosemary essential oil

2 drops Lime essential oil

Rectifying Deep Painful Chest Cough

2 drops Rosemary essential oil

2 drops Frankincense essential oil

2 drops Eucalyptus essential oil

Rectifying Dry Hacking Cough

2 drops Lemon essential oil-

2 drops Eucalyptus essential oil

2 drops Rosemary essential oil

Instructions For All Three:

1. Rub oils lightly on chest.

2. Cup hand and deeply inhale the oils from your hands for a few minutes.

3. Next, pull the neck of the shirt you are wearing over your nose and mouth. Breathe in deeply for one or two minutes until the aroma starts to dissipate. (If you feel you are not getting enough energy, take breaks and then resume).

4. The oils will penetrate into the lungs, leaving you with a cooling sensation.

5. Do this daily, as many times as you can.

Tea Remedy For Cough

1 drop Clove essential oil

1 drop lemon essential oil

80z Water

1-2 drops Honey (to ensure that the water and essential oils do not separate).

1 tablespoon of Extra virgin coconut oil (optional)

Instructions

1. Boil water. Add the honey and oils to the water. Blend in a blender at high speed for about 1 minute.

2. Towel the head and keep it over the steaming cup to enjoy the therapeutic steam.

3. Enjoy the great taste as its moves along the esophagus into the body's organs and inner tissues.

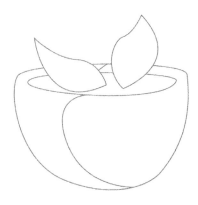

Catarrh Remedy

Catarrh is the overproduction and secretion of mucus from the throat and nose. The causes include colds, flu, bronchitis, hay fever, sinusitis and rhinitis.

1 drop Thyme essential oil

1 drop Eucalyptus essential oil

Instructions

1. In a bowl of hot water, drop the oils.

2. Drape a towel over your head

3. Inhale for 10 minutes.

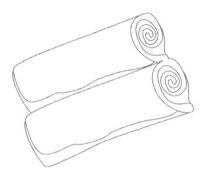

Catarrh Rub

3 drops of Eucalyptus oil

3 drops of Tea tree oil

3 drops Rosemary oil

15 ml Evening primrose oil

<u>Instructions</u>

Combine and rub on the chest and the back area.

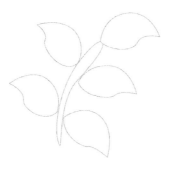

FEVER

A fever is an unusually high body temperature. It is caused by a viral or bacterial infection. Symptoms include shivering, apathy, headache, upward turning of the eyes and dullness. If a fever escalates, it could cause seizures or even delirium which could affect the brain.

Fever Massage Blend

15 ml Evening primrose oil

1 drop Rosemary essential oil

1 drop Tea Tree essential oil

2 drops Eucalyptus essential oil

2 drops Lavender essential oil

2 drops Peppermint essential oil

1 drop Black pepper essential oil

Instructions

1. Add oils together.

2. Massage the temples, top of hands, back of neck and soles of feet.

PAINS INSIDE THE BODY

Nerve Pain Oil

Nerves register pain; this is why damaged nerves are usually painful. However, aromatherapy treatments can help to speed up the healing process.

3 drops of marjoram oil

2 drops of lavender oil

4 drops of chamomile oil

3 drops of helichrysum oil (optional)

1 oz vegetable oil

Instructions

1. Combine all ingredients.

2. Apply daily for pain relief. Use as needed.

Achy Muscle Soother

2 drops Lemongrass essential oil

4 drops Ginger essential oil

4 drops Lavender essential oil

4 teaspoons Almond oil

Instructions

Combine and apply on affected areas.

Muscle Pain Massage

2 drops Lavender

2 drops Rosemary

4 teaspoons any carrier oil

Instructions

1. Combine oils and massage gently onto affected area.

Rheumatic Pain Essential Oil Blend

2 drops Lavender Essential Oil

4 drops Silver Fir Essential Oil

4 drops Ginger Essential Oil

4 teaspoons Carrier oil of choice

Instructions

Combine and apply on affected areas.

Cramp Relief EO For Muscle Pain

Muscles may hurt after a long day of work or vigorous exercise. Repeated daily activities may also tighten muscles, causing them to cramp.

12 drops Lavender essential oil

6 drops Marjoram essential Oil

4 drops Chamomile essential Oil

4 drops Ginger essential oil

2 ounces Vegetable oil

Instructions

1. Combine all ingredients.

2. Apply daily over the cramping area as often as needed

For Rheumatism & Arthritis

3 drops Chamomile

3 drops Yarrow

3 drops Lavender

3 drops Eucalyptus

8 ounces sweet-almond oil

Instructions

1. Add the essential oils to almond oil

2. Massage into affected areas.

Essential Oil Liniment For Joint Pain

Several factors cause joint pain. Injury, overuse and damage from previous injury or disease are some of these. The condition may be mild, lasting for a few hours or it may be chronic, lasting for several years. Essential oil helps to limit the inflammation that often comes with it.

8 drops Eucalyptus essential oil

8 drops Peppermint essential oil

8 drops Rosemary essential oil

4 drops Cinnamon leaf oil

4 drops Juniper berry oil

4 drops Marjoram essential oil

2 ounces Vegetable oil or vodka

Instructions

1. Mix all ingredients.

2. Every day, stir a few times for three days to disperse the oils in the alcohol.

3. This formula must not be used over a large area of the body. This is because it is stronger than the typical massage oil so make sure to use only on the painful joints

4. Use several times daily as needed.

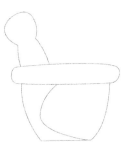

Massage Blend For Sore Joints/ Arthritis

3 drops Coriander essential oil

6 drops Roman Chamomile essential oil

4 drops Marjoram essential oil

3 drops Rosemary essential oil

1 drop Black Pepper essential oil

1 drop Ginger essential oil

2 ounces Carrier Oil of choice

Instructions

1. Blend well and store in a plastic bottle.

2. Massage daily into sore joints.

Arthritic Soaking Bath Blend

1-2 cups Bath Salt Blend

2 drops Lavender essential oil

2 drops Rosemary essential oil

4 drops Juniper berry essential oil

4 drops Cypress essential oil

Instructions

Add this blend to bath and soak for 20 to 30 minutes.

Tendonitis Relief With Essential Oil

Tendonitis is the inflammation of a tendon. It is a painful and debilitating condition caused by overuse infection or rheumatic disease. However, natural essentials oils can offer a measure of relief and quicken the healing process.

10 drops Basil essential oil

8 drops Wintergreen essential oil

6 drops Cypress essential oil

3 drops Peppermint essential oil

Instructions

1. Mix oils together, rub on location

2. Alternatively, mix with 2 tbsp of jojoba oil and massage larger areas of the body.

Abdominal Pain Care

Causes of abdominal pain include eating too fast, digestive problems or menstruation.

1 drop of Chamomile oil

1 drop of Peppermint oil

1 drop of Clove oil

5 ml Carrier oil of choice

Instructions

1. Dilute the essential oils in the carrier.

2. Massage the stomach area gently in a clockwise motion.

3. If the pain persists, seek medical advice.

Other Pain Relieving Therapies

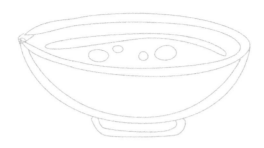

Anal Fissures Cure

These are inflamed tears around the anus caused by straining (usually caused by constipation), excessive rubbing and use of rough toilet paper.

5 drop Lavender essential oil

1 drop Lemon essential oil

Instructions

1. Add the oils to a bowl of warm water and bathe the area twice daily.

Increase Back Circulation

2 to3 drops Geranium, Citrus Bliss, Eucalyptus, Peppermint, Cypress or Lemon essential oil

Instructions

Apply topically to spinal area 2 to 3 times per day

Back Pain Inflammation Reduction

2 to 3drops Black Pepper, basil, wintergreen, bergamot or Rosemary essential oil

Instructions

Apply to spinal area topically.

EO For Neck Pain Relief

Neck pain usually affects your range of motion. Reduce the spasm and pain in your neck muscles through essential oil application.

5 drops Rosemary, peppermint, lavender or juniper essential oil

Instructions

1. Blend the oils in the palm of the hands.

2. Massage mixture into stiff or sore neck.

3. Wrap neck in a scarf for some hours.

Heal And Regenerate Tissue

1 -2 drops Frankincense, Helichrysum or Sandalwood essential oil:

Instructions

1. Apply twice or thrice daily and topically to the spinal area.

2. Have a hot compress

Eliminate Spasms And Relax Muscles

2 to3 drops Chamomile, Marjoram, AromaTouch, Lime or Roman essential oil

<u>Instructions</u>

Apply topically to the area where the spasm occurs.

Cotton Ball Remedy For Earache

An earache is usually pain in the middle or inner ear. In infants and small children, it is generally the result of irritations brought about by cleaning with a cotton swab or reactions to cleaning products. The trapped fluid puts pressure on the eardrum, causing ache.

3 drops Basil essential oil

1/2 of a cotton ball

2 to 3 drops Grapefruit essential oil

<u>Instructions</u>

1. Put the basil on a cotton ball and push it into the ear very lightly. (Do not place the oils directly into the ear as vapor from the cotton ball will get to the infected area).

2. Leave it overnight.

3. For additional relief, rub grapefruit oil behind and around the external part of the ear.

4. Place a warm cloth over the ear, while lying down.

Swab Method For Earache

2-3 drops Melrose, lavender or tea-tree essential oil

Water

Instructions

1. Dilute essential oil with warm water.

2. Swab area around the ear opening, the ear lobe and the exterior part.

Remedy For Broken Bones

Broken or fractured bones can happen anywhere in the body. Here are the essential oils that will help:

- For pain relief: Wintergreen essential oil

- For healing: Birch essential oil (bone repair), Helichrysum (nerve damage, overall tissue regeneration and repair), Cypress (circulation), Lemongrass essential oil (ligaments), White Fir (anti-inflammatory) and Marjoram (tissue rebuilding).

- For stress relief: Lavender essential oil

Instructions

1. Apply 1-2 drops topically to injured area 2- 3 times daily.

ORAL HEALTH

Simple Toothache Treatment

Toothache is usually very painful. It can be regarded as one of the worst pains caused by a minor ailment.

<u>Instructions</u>

1. Put 1 drop of clove essential oil on a cotton bud.

2. Place the cotton bud on the gum around the tooth.

2. Alternatively, place into the crevices on either side.

Toothache Essential Oil Blend

4 drops Clove bud essential oil

1 drop Orange essential oil (for flavor)

1 teaspoon Vegetable oil

Instructions

1. Add together all the ingredients and then rub a few drops onto the painful gums. Repeat frequently.

2. During an emergency, put clove bud in the most painful area of the mouth. Mash the clove gently with the teeth as it softens. By doing this, the oil is released and you can then suck on it.

3. The clove oil may be too hot for some young children. Use chamomile oil instead. Since chamomile is less effective as a pain killer, apply treatment as frequently as possible.

Massage Oil For Toothache

1 drop Lemon oil

1 drop Clove oil

3 drops Chamomile oil

5 ml vegetable oil

Instructions

1. Dilute in vegetable oil.

2. Massage the cheek and jawbone.

Tonsillitis Essential Oil Relief

Tonsillitis simply means inflammation of the tonsils. It is generally caused by viral or bacterial infection. While it may be treated via different medical procedures, essential oil basically helps to lessen the swelling and discomfort.

1 qt Water

3 drops Lemon, lavender or eucalyptus essential oil

Instructions

1. Boil water and add the essential oils. Place toweled head over hot pot of water. Breathe the aroma.

2. May also be drank as tea to relieve sore throat or used in a warm bath.

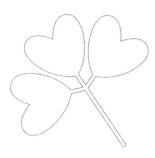

Therapeutic Mouthwash For Fresh Breath

2 drops Tea Tree essential oil

2 drops Myrrh essential oil

1 drop Peppermint essential oil

4 to 8 Ounces Distilled water

Instructions

1. Mix together in a glass or plastic PET bottle. Shake well before use.

2. Swish about 1/2 ounce in your mouth after eating as required or after brushing your teeth.

Simple Mouth Wash

2 drops Peppermint essential oil

4 drops Lemon essential oil

2 cups of Distilled water

Instructions

1. Combine oils and water. Shake before each use thoroughly.

2. Swish a mouthful for 1 to 2 minutes and spit out.

Gum Strengthener
Firm up gums and prevent gum disease.

1 drop Cinnamon

1 teaspoon of vodka

2 tablespoons of water

Instructions

1. Add the essential oil to vodka and water. Shake the mixture thoroughly.

2. Swish your toothbrush in this mixture. Brush your teeth as usual.

Remedy For Mouth Ulcers (Stomatitis)
Mouth ulcers also called stomatitis mostly occur on the tongue, inner lip, inner cheek, floor of the mouth and soft palate. It is a painful that makes chewing and eating difficult. It is caused by a variety of factors including dietary deficiencies, Candida and friction from a denture.

3 drops Myrrh essential oil

A teaspoon of Alcohol

Instructions

1. Dab directly onto the ulcer with a cotton bud. (May sting for a while but is often very effective).

2. Alternatively, dilute with half a glass of water and make into a mouthwash.

Gum Blend

10 drops Tea Tree essential oil

1 drops Peppermint essential oil

3 drops Lemon essential oil

6 drops Myrrh essential oil

1 teaspoon Almond oil

Instructions

1. Brush the teeth and rinse the mouth with mouthwash.

2. Afterwards, combine the above oils and apply a small quantity on your gums daily.

3. See your dentist if the gums or the cause of irritation do not heal.

Cold Sores & Fever Blisters

Heal your cold sores and reduce breakouts with this blend

2 drops of Roman Chamomile essential

2 drops of Eucalyptus essential oil

2 drops of Melissa essential oil

5 ml of Sweet Almond oil

Instructions

1. Mix all the ingredients very well.

2. Dab on the blister with a cotton-tip applicator.

Mouth Ulcers

Mouth ulcers are tiny open sores in the mouth, tongue, the roof of the mouth or the mucus membrane inside the cheeks and lips. While they can last from 2 days-3weeks, they heal spontaneously and leave no scar.

Instructions

1. Put 2 drops Tea Tree oil in cotton bud & apply to the ulcer.

2. Another way to address this is to make a mouthwash. Combine 2 drops of Tea Tree oil and 5ml salt to 500 ml water that has been boiled and now warm.

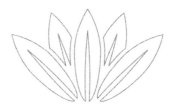

Power Mouthwash Blend
For mouth ulcer

2 drops Geranium oil

2 drops Thyme oil

2 drops Peppermint oil

2 drops Lemon oil

2 drops Tea tree oil

1 glass warm water

10 ml brandy

Instructions

1. Add all ingredients together & Use as mouthwash.

2. Swish around the mouth and spit.

Bad Breath Fighter

Bad breath is embarrassing. It could be a symptom of a root problem such as indigestion or improper toxic elimination by the liver or kidney. It could be caused by plaque buildup, decomposing food between the teeth, cigarette smoking and ingestion of strong foods such as garlic and onions.

4 drops Lavender oil

125 ml warm water

5 ml Brandy

Instructions

1. Dilute the oil in the brandy and water and use as mouthwash.

2. Swirl around the mouth after brushing and flossing. Rinse and spit out.

3. Use as needed.

Bad Breath Due To Gum Disease

2 drops Tea tree essential oil

2 drops Thyme essential oil

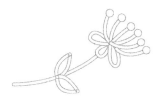

Bad Breath Due To Digestive Issues

2 drops Peppermint essential oil

A teaspoon of Brandy

2 drops Lemon essential oil

Instructions For Both Recipes

1. Dilute the essential oil in brandy. Add mixture to a glass of warm water.

2. Sip, swirl around then mouth and spit out. Do not swallow.

Chapped Lips

Chapped lips can be very painful. It is difficult to keep from licking your sore lips but this process usually increases the pain.

1 drop Chamomile oil

1 drop Neroli oil

2 drops Rose oil

2 drops Geranium oil

20 ml Aloe Vera oil

Instructions

1. Mix all the ingredients together in a roller bottle.

2. Apply to lips to ease pain and foster healing.

STOMACH RELIEF

Hiccups
Hiccups are not meant to last for a long time otherwise they can be very painful.

Instructions

1. In a brown paper bag, place 1 drop Chamomile essential oil.

2. Now, hold the bag over your nose and mouth.

3. Breathe in slowly but deeply through your nose.

Massage Oil For Diarrhea
Diarrhea is the frequent and excessive discharge of the bowel movement. It is abnormal condition that shows that something is not right with the system. It could be due to excessive food consumption, eating spicy foods, undigested vegetables, unripe fruits, eating too fast or drinking unclean water

2 drops Lavender essential oil

2 drops Geranium essential oil

2 drops Peppermint essential oil

2 drops Chamomile essential oil

2 drops Eucalyptus essential oil

10 ml Vegetable carrier oil

Instructions

1. Combine the ingredients in a dark bottle.

2. Rub over abdominal area twice a day.

Nausea Instant Therapy

The underlying cause of nausea can be physiological, psychological or even both. Reasons such as disgusting smells, hangovers, bad digestion, food poisoning, motion sickness, early pregnancy and tonsillitis could contribute to nausea.

1 drop Lavender essential oil

1 drop Peppermint essential oil

1 drop Basil essential oil

2 teaspoons (10ml) Carrier oil

Instructions

1. Mix the oils with the carrier oil.

2. Massage gently over your abdomen.

3. Before washing your hands, cup your hands over your mouth and nose and inhale slowly a few times.

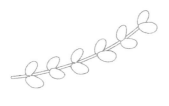

Diverticulitis Relief Blend

Individuals above the age of forty can develop diverticulitis when there is continuous pressure against weakened tissue. Drinking Aloe Vera juice 2 or 3 times a day can promote healing.

2 drops Rosemary essential oil

1 drop Peppermint essential oil

1 drop Clove essential oil

1 drop Chamomile essential oil

1 teaspoon (5ml) Vegetable carrier oil

Instructions

1. Blend oils together.

2. Use as massage oil to relieve the discomfort.

Diarrhea Capsule Blend

2 drops Oregano essential oil

3 drops Mountain savory essential oil

4drops Lemon essential oil

3 drops of vegetable oil

Instructions

1. Blend oils and the add 2-3 drops of the blend to the vegetable oil in a 00 size capsule.

2. Swallow, twice daily.

Motion Sickness Relief

Motion sickness can be relieved and also prevented by the following blend.

10 drops Peppermint essential oil

10 drops Ginger essential oil

10 drops Roman Chamomile essential oil

Instructions

1. Blend all the essential oils in a dark bottle.

2. Put a few drops on a tissue and inhale. You can also make use of a personal inhaler.

3. Inhale about 30 to 60 minutes before embarking on a journey and every 15 to 30 minutes when on the way.

Sniff Remedy To Treat Motion Sickness

2 drops lavender or bergamot essential oil

Instructions

1. Add the essential oil to a handkerchief and sniff.

2. Get enough fresh air.

Bladder Infection Sitz Bath

5 drops lavender oil

5 drops rosemary oil

Instructions

1. Add the essential oils to a hot bath

2. Sit for 5 to10 minutes in a tub with the hot water up to the waist.

3. Switch to a tub of cold water for at 1-2 minute and do 2 to 5 rounds.

Bladder Infection Oil

8 drops juniper berry or cypress oil

2 drops fennel oil

6 drops tea tree oil

6 drops bergamot oil

2 ounces vegetable oil

Instructions

1. Combine all ingredients. Massage once a day over the bladder area.

2. For prevention, add 1 tablespoon of this mixture to your bath.

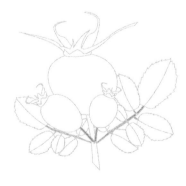

DIGESTIVE ISSUES

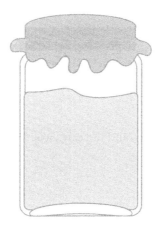

Constipation Relief Recipe

You are constipated when bowel movements are fewer than 3 to 4 in a week. Implement this rectifying procedure:

5 drops Peppermint essential oil

10 drops Lemon essential oil

15 drops Rosemary essential oil

30 ml Jojoba oil

Instructions

1. Blend oils together.

2. Massage in a clockwise motion over the abdominal area thrice a day.

3. Do this treatment daily or at least two times a week.

Stomach Massage For Indigestion

2 drops Cinnamon

6 drops Mandarin

4 drops Peppermint

2 tablespoons carrier oil

Instructions

1. Mix the essential oils and the carrier oil well.

2. Massage onto stomach.

Heartburn Relief

Heartburn is an uncomfortable burning pain in the lower chest. It often occurs after a meal.

2 drops Eucalyptus oil

1 drop Peppermint oil

2 drops Fennel oil

1 teaspoon (5ml) Grape seed oil

Instructions

1. Dilute the essential oils in the carrier oil

2. Rub the upper abdominal area with this mixture.

Gerd Abdominal Rub

2 drop Eucalyptus essential oil

1 drop Peppermint essential oil

2 drop Fennel essential oil

Grapeseed oil 1 teaspoon (5ml)

Instructions

1. Mix the essential oils with the carrier oil.

2. Rub on the upper abdominal area anytime you have burning pain in your chest.

Acid Reflux /Gerd Drink

1 drop of Lemon essential oil

1 drop of Peppermint essential oil

12-16 oz. of drinking water

Instructions

1. Add the oil to your water and drink all through the day.

2. For an intense episode, add 3 drops of Lemon essential oil to a small glass of warm water and drink.

Indigestion Digestive Stimulant

3 drops Roman Chamomile essential oil

3 drops Ginger essential oil

5 drops Bergamot essential oil

1 ounce Grapeseed oil

Instructions

1. Blend the oils in a bottle. Massage the stomach and the intestinal area rubbing in a clockwise motion.

2. Alternatively, add a drop of Lemon essential oil to a cup of Chamomile tea and drink.

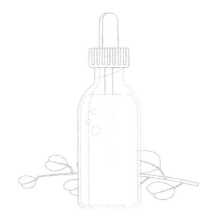

Flatulence (Gas) Massage Blend

This massage blend is recommended when flatulence is accompanied by pain and discomfort.

2 drops Peppermint essential oil

3drops Rosemary essential oil

1 drop Clove essential oil

1 drop Chamomile essential oil

1 teaspoon (5ml) Olive oil

Instructions

1. Rub the blend over your abdominal area twice daily.

Flatulence (Gas) Relief Capsule

1-2 drops of Ginger essential oil

1-2 drops of Lavender essential oil

3-4 drops of vegetable oil

Instructions

1. Add either of these essential oils to the vegetable oil in a capsule.

2. Take the capsule 15 to 30 minutes before intake of any food that can cause flatulence.

Bloating Remedy

2 drops Lemongrass or Cypress essential oil

4 drops Lemon or Grapefruit essential oil

1 tablespoon Grapeseed oil

Instructions

1. Properly blend oils together.

2. Massage the swollen area with upward motions, 2- 3 times daily.

3. In addition, add1-2 drops of Lemon essential oil to a glass of water and drink 3 times daily.

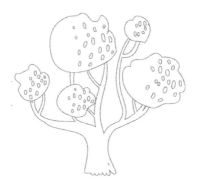

RECIPES FOR HAIR CARE

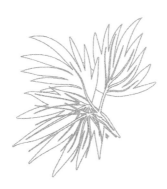

Remedy For Light Dandruff

Dandruff occurs when excessive skin oils and cells die and flake off in unusually large quantities. Although not a serious condition, it is often embarrassing.

2 to 3 drops Melaleuca or tea tree

Any high quality shampoo

Instructions

Add oil to shampoo and use.

Essential Oil Blend For Heavy Dandruff

1 teaspoon any carrier oil

4 drops Lavender essential oil

4 drops Lemon essential oil

4 drops Melaleuca essential oil

4 drops Rosemary essential oil

Instructions

1. Blend and massage into the scalp every night and then cover with shower cap.

2. Shampoo it out the following morning.

Anti-Flaking Treatment

Break the cycle of damaged scalp and flaking caused by substandard dandruff shampoos by using the following:

4 -6 drops Birch, Wintergreen or Rosemary

1/2 ounce Shampoo

Instructions

1. Mix the oil into the shampoo. Apply1 inch partings in the hair and then rub mixture into scalp.

2. Let it stay on for 5-7 minutes and then apply regular shampoo and conditioning.

Mild Hair Loss Remedy

1 or 2 drops of Rosemary essential oil

Instructions

1. Mix together essential oil to shampoo

2. Use it every day to stimulate follicle

Serious Hair Loss Remedy

3 drops Rosemary essential oil

5 drops Lavender essential oil

4 drops Cypress essential oil

4 drops Clary Sage essential oil

10 drops Sandalwood

Instructions

Combine all ingredients and pour in your hair shampoo.

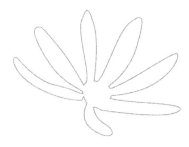

Dandruff & Scaly Scalp Blend

2 drops Atlas cedarwood essential oil

2 drops Rosemary essential oil

2 drops tea tree oil essential oil

2 drops Lavender essential oil

1/2 ounce Jojoba

Instructions

Combine and apply to scalp

Hair Growth/ Softener Recipe

2 drops Thyme essential oil

3 drops Rosemary essential oil

2 drops Cedar essential oil

1 ounce Grapeseed

1 tbsp Jojoba

Instructions

1. Combine ingredients into a tight bottle.

2. Massage into your scalp every night.

3. Rinse the next morning in cool water and shampoo.

3. Use thrice a week for oily hair and once for normal.

Wood Haven Beard Oil

Oil and beautify your beard, moisturize the dry skin underneath it and smell really wonderful!

3 drops peppermint essential oil

1/4oz sweet almond oil

5 drops tea tree oil essential oil

3/4oz jojoba oil

Instructions

1. Combine in 1 oz bottle, shake well, dap on your fingers and rub on your beards.

2. Best use after a shower when your beard is washed and your skin is fresh.

Minty Fresh Beard Oil

1/2oz sweet almond oil

2 drops tea tree oil

5 drops peppermint oil

2 drops orange oil

1/2oz jojoba oil

3/4oz jojoba oil

Instructions

1. Combine in 1 oz bottle, shake well, dap on your fingers and rub on your beards.

2. Best use after a shower when your beard is washed and your skin is

fresh.

Fall Face Foliage Beard Oil

3/4oz sweet almond oil

2 drops tea tree oil

2 drops cinnamon cassia oil

2 drops orange oil

1/4oz jojoba oil

Instructions

1. Combine in 1 oz bottle, shake well, dap on your fingers and rub on your beards.

2. Best use after a shower when your beard is washed and your skin is fresh.

FOOT AND LEG CARE

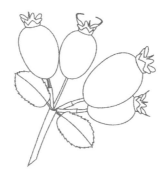

Simple Foot Powder Blend

2 drops Thyme essential oil

2 drops Tea Tree essential oil

5 drops Rosemary essential oil

5 oz Talc Powder

Instructions

1. Place oils in powder. Shake thoroughly and let it sit for 24 hours. Before using on your feet, shake again. Use daily.

2. Dust on your feet after showering. Be sure to spread your toes.

No More Dry Cracked Heels

10 drops Geranium essential oil

10 drops Melaleuca essential oil

10 drops Peppermint essential oil

1 tablespoon Virgin Coconut Oils

Instructions

1. Blend together. Apply topically on area every morning and evening.

2. Cover with socks

Food Bath Blend (for tired feet)

4 drops Grapefruit essential oil

4 drops Myrtle essential oil

3 drops Cajeput essential oil

4 drops Spearmint essential oil

1 teaspoon Sesame, Almond or Hazelnut carrier oil

Instructions

1. Blend all ingredients and add to a basin of warm water. Swirl around and then soak in your feet.

2. Relax for about 15 minutes.

Foot Odor Remedy

2-3 drops Lavender

Basin of lukewarm water

Instructions

1. Add oil to bath and then place feet (safe for blistered and cracked feet as well) in it for 10- 15 minutes.

Calluses And Corns Essential Oil Blend

Although calluses are generally painless, they tend to be painful on the bottom of feet where they occur due to poorly fitting shoes. Corns occur above the toe joints and they can cause a lot of discomfort as well.

6 drops Myrrh essential oil

4 drops Vanilla essential oil

12 drops Lavender essential oil

2 ounces Sweet almond

Instructions

1. Mix together in a bottle, shaking well to mix.

2. Massage into the affected area to soften calluses and corns. Apply daily.

Gout Relief Blend

This blend is effective for the common gout that comes with intense pain and redness of the big toe.

10 drops Frankincense essential oil

10 drops Basil essential oil

Instructions

1. Mix the oils together in a dark bottle.

2. Apply 2-3 drops of the blend to the painful area then cover with hot compress.

3. Repeat 2 or 3 times per day

Anti-Fungus Blend For Athletic Foot

Sweaty feet that are cloistered in socks and shoes are the leading cause of Athlete's foot. Such moist environments attract fungus.

12 drops Tea tree essential oil

8 drops Geranium essential oil

3 drops Thyme essential oil

1 tablespoon Tincture of benzoin

2 ounces Apple cider vinegar

2 drops Myrrh essential oil (optional)

Instructions

1. Combine all ingredients. Shake well before use.

2. Use as wash daily or as often as needed or dab on afflicted area.

Essential Oil Blend For Bone Spurs

Bone spurs (osteophytes) is simply an added bone growth to a normal bone area. This condition usually occurs after an injury as the body attempts to repair itself. Common activities like running, dancing and even wearing tight shoes can cause bone spurs.

4 drops Wintergreen essential oil

4 drops Eucalyptus essential oil

4 drops Marjoram essential oil

4 drops Cypress essential oil

4 drops Helichrysum essential oil

4 drops Peppermint essential oil

4 drops Frankincense essential oil

10 drops Coconut oil carrier

Instructions

1. Mix ingredients and apply to affected area twice daily until the bone spur gone.

2. Continue another 2 weeks. Wrap with a warm cloth to speed up results and then wrap with plastic bag and extra towel to keep heat in.

Alternative Bone Spur Solution

5 drops Eucalyptus essential oil

5 drops Marjoram essential oil

5 drops Cypress essential oil

5 drops Lavender essential oil

5 drops Thyme essential oil

5 drops Basil essential oil

30 drops Coconut carrier oil -

Instructions

1. Mix ingredients and apply to affected area twice daily until the bone spur gone.

2. Continue for 2 weeks. Wrap with a warm cloth to speed up results and then wrap with plastic bag and extra towel to keep heat in. Reported results took between 2 weeks to 3 months.

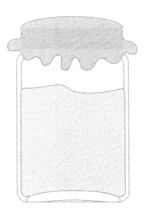

Athletic Foot Fungal Powder

14 drops Lemon eucalyptus or tea tree essential oil

8 drops Geranium essential oil

5 drops Sage essential oil

1 drops Peppermint essential oil

1/4 cup Cornstarch

Instructions

1. Place the cornstarch in a plastic bag. Gently sprinkle in the essential oils, evenly distributing them through the powder.

2. Next, close the bag and then toss the powder. This will break up any formed clumps. Store the powder in a glass or ceramic container or a sealed plastic bag. A perforated lidded shake bottle will even make dispensing easier to achieve. Use powder once daily or as often as needed.

Edema (Swollen Legs, Feet, Ankles, Arms)

This condition occurs as a result of excess fluid in the body tissues at the affected areas. The following blend will strengthen the capillary walls and enhance the drainage of blood.

3 drops Cypress essential oil

5 drops Lemon essential oil

1 tablespoon Grape- seed oil

Instructions

1. Mix oils together and use to massage the affected area. Use upward motions.

2. Repeat 2 to 3 times every day.

COMMON CHILDREN AILMENTS

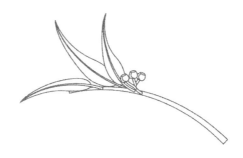

Relief For Prickly Heat Rash

Use this combination for babies two years and under. Older children will require double of the measurement.

2 drops Lavender essential oil

1/4 cup Baking Soda

Instructions

1. Mix the two ingredients together then add to bath water.

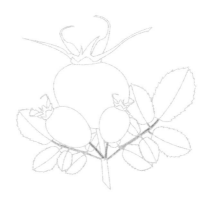

Chicken Pox
For young children

10 drops lavender

10 drops Roman Chamomile

4 oz calamine lotion

Instructions

1. Dilute oils in calamine lotion.

2. Mix well and apply over body two times daily

Kids' Flu Fighter
1 drop Cypress, lemon or Melaleuca

1 Tbsp. bath gel base

Instructions

Dilute in a bath or diffuse

Colds And Runny Nose Massage
1 drop Lavender, Tea Tree, Thyme or Niaouli essential oil

1 oz carrier oil

Instructions

Dilute and use for massaging baby's or toddler's chest or back.

Constipation No -More

For young children

1- 2 drops orange, mandarin or ginger essential oil

2tbs fractionated coconut oil

Instructions

Dilute and massage a little on the feet.

Kids' Cold Cure

10 drops Lavender

10 drops Eucalyptus

10 drops Tea Tree

Instructions

1. Combine all oils. Put 3 drops of mixture in a diffuser at bedtime.

2. For heavy congestion, put 2 drops of the mixture on cotton piece and tuck it inside the child's pillowcase at night.

3. Put 2 to 5 drops in a bath. The steam will help to clear the nasal passages and help your child to rest.

Bruises Treatment

1drop Lavender

1drop Geranium

1 oz or 2tbsp carrier oil

Instructions

Dilute and apply to the bruise.

Sunburn Eliminator

5 drops lavender

1 tsp aloe Vera

Instructions

Dilute oil and apply over sunburned area.

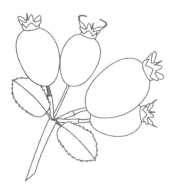

Minor Burns Care For Kids

1. Cool the skin for 10 minutes by immersing the burned skin in water.

2. If the skin isn't broken, apply 2 drops lavender essential oil directly on the burned area.

3. If the skin is broken, apply 2 drops of lavender around the burned area. Afterwards, put 5 drops of diluted lavender oil on a cold, dry cloth and then hold it over the area of the burn.

Cuts And Scrapes Care For Kids

5 drops lavender

5 drops Malaleuca

1 drop Lavender

Instructions

1. Dilute oils in a small bowl of warm water.

2. Use the diluted water to clean the cut.

3. Apply 1 drop lavender essential oil to band- aid

4. Use it to cover the wound.

Mouth Alcer Treatment

Myrrh essential oil is extremely bitter especially for children so it is best to add Peppermint, mandarin or Fennel oil to this mixture.

2 drops Myrrh essential oil

1 drops Peppermint essential oil

1 teaspoon Alcohol

Instructions

1. Using a cotton-bud, dab straight onto the ulcer.

2. Alternatively, dilute with half a glass of water and make into a mouthwash.

Essential Oil Solution For Nose Bleeds

This condition is very common with children. Helichrysum essential oil does not interfere with blood thinning medication.

2- 3 drops Helichrysum essential oil

Instructions

1. Apply oil to bleeding nostrils. Apply externally or internally using tissue saturated with helichrysum. The bleeding stops faster with internal application.

Bronchitis Relief For Children

25 drops of Myrtle essential oil

10 drops of Eucalyptus radiata essential oil

10 drops of Thyme linalool essential oil

10 drops Niaouli of essential oil

Instructions

1. Combine ingredients.

2. Drop 10 drops of the combination in a bowl of very hot water. Let the steam permeate the air.

3. When this steam is inhaled, it kills off the germs in the naval cavities, bronchial tubes and trachea.

3. Another way to use this is to simply place some drops of the mixture on a tissue and inhale.

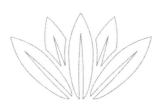

Grazes No- More

Children will always run around and may hurt themselves. Protect them from infection when grazes occur.

Instructions

1. Take out the splinter.

2. Bath all dirt thoroughly by using 10 drops lavender, tea tree, lemon or Eucalyptus in a bowl of warm water.

3. Let the damaged skin remain open in the fresh air. If there is danger of re-infection, make sure you cover-up.

Itchy Relief Repellent

Get rid of all annoying itches with this natural repellent.

Suitable for children 2 years + old

2 oz jojoba/coconut oil

10 drops neem oil

10 drops Lavender essential oil

10 drops Lemon essential oil

10 drops Thyme essential oil

10 drops Geranium essential oil

Instructions

Mix all the ingredients and store in a bottle.

HEADACHES

A headache is simply a pain in the head but the severity of the discomfort varies to a great extent. Headaches are symptomatic. The underlying cause could be stress, tension, fatigue, allergies or blocked sinuses. Others include drug overuse, adverse reaction to medication and seasonal changes.

Fast Fix Remedy

3 drops lavender essential oils

2 drops peppermint essential oils

Instructions

1. Add oils to fold-up tissue.

2. Inhale slowly and deeply in 3 long breaths.

3. Repeat three times.

For Mild Tension Headache

2-3 drops Peppermint essential oil

Instructions

Rub on the forehead, temples and back of neck.

For Severe Headache

1. Apply remedy for mild tension headache.

2. Compress the aforementioned areas with a clean, damp towel and rest for a few minutes.

3. Repeat as often as needed. A few drops may be added to the towel to speed up the help.

4. Keep oils away from eyes.

Anti- Headache Blend

1 drop Peppermint oil

3 drops Lavender oil

3 drops Jojoba oil

1 drop Bergamot oil

Instructions

1. Mix oils and massage around the temples or into the base of the skull.

Migraine Headache Hand Soak

5 drops Lavender essential oil

5 drops Ginger essential oil

1 quart (about 110°F) Hot water

Instructions

1. Add the essential oils to the hot water.

2. Soak hands for about 3 minutes.

3. This therapy may be done repeatedly.

Tension/ Nervous Headache Mix

1 drop Clary sage oil

3 drops of Lavender oil

2 drops of Jojoba oil

1 drop Chamomile oil

Instructions

1. Mix oils and massage around the temples or into the base of the skull.

Headache Balm

1 tablespoon Beeswax, grated

1/4 cup Shea Butter

1/4 teaspoon (or 1 capsule) Vitamin E

1 tablespoon Grapeseed oil

8 drops Lavender essential oil

1 drop Chamomile essential oil

1 drop Jasmine essential oil

Instructions

1. Place the beeswax, Shea butter & grapeseed oil in a double boiler over a low heat until melted.

2. Remove from heat; add the essential oils and the vitamin E. Pour into a dark glass jar and store in a cool, dark place.

3. Rub onto back of your neck and your temples to ease pain and soothe tension

SKIN BLEMISHES/COSMETIC PROBLEMS

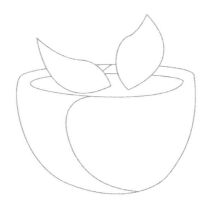

Sunburn Soother

20 drops of lavender oil

1 tablespoon vinegar

200 IU vitamin E oil

4 ounces aloe Vera juice

Instructions

1. Combine all the ingredients. Shake thoroughly before using.

2. Store in a spritzer bottle and use as needed.

3. Keeping the spray refrigerated provides extra relief due to the coolness.

Aromatherapy Treatment For Acne

It's ok to have one or two pimples now and then but when breakouts are frequent; this blend can be very helpful.

3 drops Geranium essential oil

7 drops Tea Tree or Lemongrass essential oil -

10 drops Lavender essential oil

Jojoba oil or Aloe Vera gel - 30ml

Instructions

1. Mix jojoba oil with essential oils in a dark glass bottle.

2. Apply a little quantity to affected areas of the skin twice a day. Avoid eyes, lips and nose.

3. Results will appear if used consistently for a few weeks.

Blemish Blocker

Dab a little of this highly effective mix on your pimple; do not use too often because it may dry out your skin

10 drops Lemon

10 drops Lavender

10 drops Tea Tree

Instructions

1. Combine oils in a dark glass container.

2. Use a cotton swab to apply tiny amounts to skin blemishes.

3. *Note:* although lemon is not usually applied neat, unlike lavender and tea tree, it is safe for spot-treating" purpose in this preparation.

Intensive Blemish Treatment

12 drops tea tree oil

1/2 teaspoon of powdered Oregon grape root, powdered

800 units vitamin E (optional)

A few drops of water

Instructions

1. Add together the herb powder and essential oil, stirring to make a paste.

2. Apply directly as a mask on the blemished area.

3. Allow the paste to dry and remain on your skin for 20- 30 minutes, then rinse off.

Stretch Marks Treatment Lotion

3 drops Lavender essential oil

3 drops Frankincense essential oil

3 drops Geranium essential oil

3 drops Helichrysum essential oil

1 ounce Virgin coconut oil

Instructions

1. Use this blend as body lotion on affected areas.

Itchy Skin Recipe

5 drops Lavender essential oil

3 drops Tea Tree essential oil

2 drops Frankincense essential oil

2 ounces Witch hazel

Instructions

1. Fill a 2 ounce spray bottle halfway with witch hazel, add the essential oils, shake together then fill remaining space with witch hazel.

2. Apply this mixture on itchy skin.

Age Spots Remedy

2 drops Frankincense essential oil

2 drops Lavender essential oil

2 drops Myrrh essential oil

10ml Extra virgin coconut oil

Instructions

1. Mix the ingredients together and apply topical at least once a day.

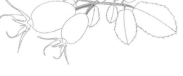

Wrinkles And Mature Skin Blend

15 drops Lavender

5 drops Frankincense

5 drops Carrot seed

5 drops Neroli

2 ounces Jojoba oil

Instructions

1. Mix ingredients together in a dark bottle.

2. Massage the affected areas as needed.

Gentle Wart Removal

Eliminate warts and prevent future outbreaks

1 drop Lemon essential oil (per wart)

Apply undiluted to the affected area directly. Do this several times a day for at 4-5 weeks.

Stretch Marks Cocoa Butter Cream

4 drops Neroli essential oil

1 ounces Avocado oil

3 ounces Cocoa butter (deodorized)

Instructions

1. Melt cocoa butter in a double boiler then stir in avocado oil.

2. Pour the mixture in a bowl to cool then add the essential oil.

3. Transfer to a 4 ounce jar with a lid and use as body cream.

4. Store in the refrigerator to avoid the growth of mold.

Aromatherapy For Scars

Reduce the visibility of scars that may have developed from surgeries, scrapes and cuts with this blend.

4 drops Lavender essential oil

6 drops Helichrysum essential oil

1 ounce Rosehip seed oil

Instructions

1. Mix this combination in a bottle.

2. Start using daily on the cut once it is sealed shut (this could be after a few days). Apply the blend over the scab and the immediate area. Do not remove the scabs on the surface. Picking or removing scabs will lead to scarring.

3. If you had a surgery, start applying the blend once the staples and sutures are removed.

4. This blend can also be used on old scars but it takes 3-6 months to get results.

Treatment For Cracked Skin

The Lavender oil in this blend will help to fight infected cracks in the skin. You should also endeavor to drink adequate water daily to keep your body hydrated.

10 drops Lavender essential oil

5 drops Neroli essential oil

5 drops Helichrysum essential oil

1 ounce Lotion

Instructions

1. Mix the essential oils with 1 ounce of your body lotion.

2. Apply as many times as necessary daily. It will stimulate healing of cracks and the regeneration of new cells.

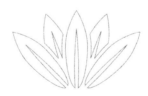

SKIN CARE

Easy Facial Toner

5 drops Lavender

5 drops Yarrow

4 oz. Springwater

Instructions

1. Combine all the ingredients. Use as a facial toner.

2. Alternately, add only the essential oils to a simple moisturizer or lotion.

Sunscreen Recipe

30 drops Helichrysum essential oil

30 drops Lavender essential oil

Fractionated Coconut oil

Instructions

1. Add the essential oils to 2 ounce spray bottle then fill up the bottle with fractionated coconut oil.

2. Shake and spray on your body as sunscreen.

Oily Skin Remedy

3 drops Geranium essential oil

3 drops Grapefruit essential oil

3 drops Lavender essential oil

30ml Evening primrose carrier oil

Instructions

1. Mix the ingredients in a glass bottle.

2. Apply a little quantity to your face every day.

Sun Spots Aromatherapy Remedy

5 drops Frankincense essential oil

5 drops Lavender essential oil

Distilled water

Instructions

1. Mix these essential oils with water in a 2 ounce spray bottle.

2. Spray this mixture on your skin before rubbing on your sunscreen or moisturizer every other day.

Dry Skin Moisturizer

7 drops Geranium essential oil

10 drops Sandalwood essential oil

3 drops Rosewood essential oil

5 drops Ylang Ylang essential oil

2 ounces Carrier oil

Instructions

1. Mix all ingredients together in a bottle.

2. Apply 4 - 6 drops of this blend to dry area twice a day.

Oily Skin Steam Bath
This recipe is good for stimulating facial skin.

4 drops Lemon essential oil

6 drops Juniper Berry essential oil

4 drops Cypress essential oil

Instructions

1. Add the oils above to a bowl of hot water.

2. Bend over the bowl; drape a towel over your head and the bowl to prevent the escape of steam.

3. Hold this position for 5-10 minutes then use tepid water to rinse your face and pat dry.

Skin Firming Recipe For Flabby Skin

If your skin is sagging after weight loss, restore elasticity and improve blood flow with this recipe.

8 drops Patchouli essential oil

5 drops Cypress essential oil

5 drops Geranium essential oil

1 drop Sandalwood essential oil

1/2 teaspoon Jojoba oil

Instructions

1. Mix these ingredients together to make a soothing skin serum.

2. Massage affected areas before bed at night and sometimes in the morning.

SKIN INJURIES AND PROBLEMS

Cuts Spray

To reduce the risk of infection

6 drops eucalyptus oil

12 drops tea tree oil

6 drops of lemon oil

2 oz distilled water

Instructions

1. Combine all the ingredients, shaking well before each use.

2. Dispense as needed from a spray bottle. Use on minor cuts, burns or abrasions to speed healing and prevent infection.

Boils Treatment

Boils can appear on different parts of the body and can sometimes be associated with fever and fatigue.

2 drops Tea tree essential oil

2 drops Lavender essential oil

1 drops Juniper essential oil

Instructions

1. Dilute the essential oils in 200 ml of hot water.

2. Bathe the infected area twice daily with this mixture.

3. For severe inflammation, add 1drop of Chamomile essential oil.

Blisters

Blisters are brought about by fluid accumulation underneath the skin. They are painful swelling on the skin. Once the blister bursts, the exposed tissue beneath could become infected. Injury, burning, an insect sting, scalding or chafing could result in blisters.

1 drop of tea tree oil or lavender

Instructions

1. Simply apply oil onto the blister.

2. Carefully but thoroughly pat in.

Ringworm Treatment

The Melaleuca and Thyme in this blend are effective against fungal infections while the Lavender will aid healing of the skin.

30 drops Melaleuca essential oil

30 drops Thyme essential oil

30 drops Lavender essential oil

Instructions

1. Apply 2-3 drops of this combination topically on infected area 3 times daily for 10 to 12 days

Emergency Burn Wash/Compress

5 drops lavender oil

1 pint water, about 50°F

Instructions

1. Add the oil to the water, stirring well to disperse the oil.

2. Soak a soft cloth in the water and then apply to the burn. Let it stay for 5-10 minutes. Repeat process twice.

3. Alternatively, immerse the burned area directly in the water for 5 minutes.

Scabies Aromatherapy Treatment

4 drops Peppermint essential oil

4 drops Lavender essential oil

1 teaspoon Sweet Almond oil

Instructions

1. Apply this blend to itching areas 2-3 times a day, after a bath.

2. Wash clothing of affected person at high temperature. Spray pillows, mattresses, couches with a mixture of 5% lavender, 5% white camphor and 90% alcohol. Wear a mask while spraying to avoid inhaling.

Bruise

A bruise is a skin discoloration that occurs when blood leaks from damaged blood vessels into the surrounding tissues under the skin. Bruises usually heal naturally but you could use the remedy below for an extra boost.

5 drops Calendula oil

2 drops Fennel oil

1 drop Cypress oil

10 ml Grape seed oil

Instructions

1. Dilute essential oils in carrier oil and massage the affected area.

Eczema And Dermatitis Treatment

This blend will relieve itching, sooth the skin and also stimulate healing.

5 drops Helichrysum essential oil

3 drops Melaleuca essential oil

10 drops Lavender essential oil

5 drops Myrrh essential oil

1 teaspoon Extra virgin coconut oil

Instructions

1. Mix together and apply topically on affected area daily.

Cuts And Wounds Antiseptic Cream

20 drops Lavender Essential Oil

15 drops Tea Tree Essential Oil

15 drops Geranium Essential Oil

43 ml Base Cream

Instructions

1. Add the Base Cream to a fill 2/3 of 50 ml dark colored glass jar.

2. Add essential oils, mixing with a spoon. Fill jar

3. Use directly onto injury, cover with bandage for quicker healing.

Warts Remedy

12 drops Lemon essential oil

4 drops Bergamot FCF essential oil

4 drops Tea Tree essential oil

3 drops Cypress essential oil

4 drops Thyme essential oil

1 tablespoon Jojoba oil

Instructions

1. Blend together in a dark glass bottle.

2. Apply 2 drops of this blend to the wart then cover with a Band-Aid.

3. Do this once a day for 2 weeks.

Note: Use 2 teaspoons of jojoba oil if using on the elderly or children.

Small Open Wound Bleeding

Bleeding should always be taken seriously, regardless of what kind it is. An adult usually has about 5 liter of blood. Even the loss of 1 liter can be fatal.

1 drop Chamomile oil

1 drop Geranium oil

1 drop Lemon oil

1 drop Tea Tree oil

Instructions

1. Combine and apply as a compress

Shingles Relief With Essential Oil

Shingles is a skin rash caused by an inflammation of the nerve and skin. It is caused by the same virus that causes chicken-pot.

30 drops Melaleuca essential oil

30 drops Eucalyptus essential oil

30 drops Lavender essential oil

Instructions

1. Mix and add to a 4-ounce spray bottle. Fill it with fractionated coconut oil. Shake thoroughly before spraying.

2. Spray directly to affected area as often as needed to deal with the pain.

Anti- Abscess Compress

An abscess is typically caused by bacteria and forms around a hair follicle. Generally, it is a pus-filled cavity where the skin becomes red and swollen and later develops into a throbbing elevated lump.

2 drops Tea Tree essential oil

2 drops Lavender essential oil

2 drops Chamomile essential oil

Instructions

Combine and apply to the area of swelling twice daily.

Bed Sores (Pressure Ulcers)

Bedsores or pressure ulcers are injuries that often develop from continuous pressure applied to the skin when in a limited area. People who are confined to a chair or bed for an extended period usually experience this problem.

10 drops Lavender essential oil

6 drops Helichrysum essential oil

6 drops Myrrh essential oil

4 drops Geranium essential oil

4 drops Melaleuca essential oil

2 tbs. FCO or EVCO carrier oil

Instructions

Apply topically thrice a day

Boils

Boils are abscesses usually found at the buttocks or underarms. Fever and fatigue can be associated with boils as well.

2 drops Tea tree oil

2 drops Lavender oil

1 drop Juniper oil

200 ml hot water

Instructions

1. Dilute the essential oils in the hot water.

2. For severe inflammation, add 1 drop Chamomile oil.

3. Bathe the area two times daily.

4. Alternatively, apply undiluted tea tree or lavender oil to the area using a cotton bud.

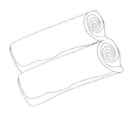

LOWER BLOOD PRESSURE

1 drop Ylang-ylang

2 drops of Clary-Sage

Instructions

Place these 3 drops on a tissue and inhale.

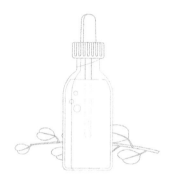

EYE CARE

Dark circles Eliminator

1 drop Roman Chamomile essential oil

1 drop Lavender essential oil

30mls Aloe Vera gel or other lotion/cream

Instructions

1. Mix the essential oils properly with aloe vera gel.

2. Once a day, cleanse and dry the face then rub the blend very gently below and above the eye socket.

3. Avoid contact with eyelids or eyelashes so you will not get some in your eyes.

Sty (Eyelid Swelling) Remedy

Sty is a temporal swelling on the eyelid. It can develop on the outside as a red sore or itchy spot, which swells and then forms a yellow or pink head. An internal sty is even more painful. The yellowish head is only noticeable when the eyelid is lifted.

Lavender or chamomile essential oil

Instructions

Dab with cotton wool 2-3 times daily

Compress Remedy For Sty

1 drop Chamomile essential oil

10 ml rosewater

Instructions

1. Add together and boil.

 2. Once cooled, place in a container and shake thoroughly.

3. Strain through a coffee filter and then use the strained mixture to make the compress.

Conjunctivitis Compress

Conjunctivitis is an infection of the conjunctiva. It can be caused by viruses, bacteria, sand, dust or smoke. Symptoms include redness, itching, irritation, burning and tearing.

1 drop Chamomile oil

5 ml Witch hazel

30 ml Rosewater

Instructions

1. Combine ingredients and leave for 7-9 hours.

2. Strain through a paper coffee filter.

3. Use as a compress on the closed eyelids.

Homemade Bugs Repellent

19 drops Lemon essential oil

25 drops Cajeput essential oil

13 drops Cedarwood essential oil

19 drops Geranium essential oil

2 oz Sweet almond oil

Instructions

1. Mix all the essential oils in a recyclable Plastic bottle.

2. Add the almond oil and Shake until thoroughly blended.

3. Apply thinly to exposed skin as needed.

Insect Repellent Spray

2 ounces distilled water

1.5 ounces witch hazel or vodka

25 drops peppermint oil

30 drops citronella oil

15 drops tea tree oil

1 teaspoon of jojoba oil (optional but if you add this, add only 1 oz of witch hazel or vodka)

<u>Instructions</u>

1. Add the vodka or witch hazel to a 4 oz clean spray bottle filled with distilled or boiled water.

2. Add the essential oils and shake thoroughly. Spray onto clothing and/or exposed skin but avoid the eyes and mucous membranes.

3. Reapply as needed. Store it in a dark bottle and away from sunlight or heat. This makes 4 ounces

Gnat And Chigger Bites Remedy

1 teaspoon Cider vinegar

3 drops Thyme essential oil

<u>Instructions</u>

1. Clean bitten area with warm soapy water, rinse and dry.

2. Combine the oil and vinegar and dab on affected area for relief.

Mosquito And Other Minor Insect Bites

1-3 drops Lavender, peppermint or tea tree essential oil

<u>Instructions</u>

1. For relief from itching, dab oil topically on affected area.

2. Repeat every 1-2 hours if necessary.

3. For very sensitive skin and for young children, dilute essential oil with a carrier oil

4. *Note:* Chamomile essential oils can reduce swelling and inflammation

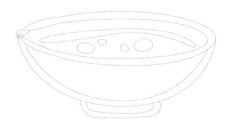

Bee Stings & Serious Insect Bites Remedy

<u>Instructions</u>

1. Remove the stinger first.

2. Then apply lavender or Roman chamomile as above.

3. Apply a cold compress over bitten area, changing regularly.

4. Do NOT use ice as it could cause damage the skin if the ice gets accidentally frozen.

5. Seek immediate medical assistance if allergic to bee stings or others.

Dog Bite Relief Blend

If there is no broken skin, clean the area and apply 1-2 drops of tea tree oil topically.

1. for puncture wound:

- Clean the area. Dilute 1 to 2 drops of Frankincense EO with carrier oil and apply topically.

   - Bandage and treat twice per day for 2 to 3 days.

2. for open wounds with torn flesh:

-Stop the bleeding using Helichrysum and pressure.

-Clean the area and then topically apply melaleuca and frankincense.

3. *Note:* If skin is damaged to the point where stitches are required or there is danger of damaged bones, tendons, ligaments or nerves, seek immediate professional medical assistance. Additionally, if there is risk of rabies, the animal should be captured if possible.

EMOTIONAL WELL BEING

Certain essential oil blends help to balance our moods and energize our bodies and spirit. Many of them can be created easily.

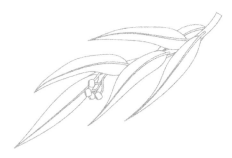

Confidence Booster

When you feel confident, it is easier to tackle tasks and challenges more effectively. This blend will give you the needed emotional support to strengthen your confidence.

10 drops Orange essential oil

10 drops Grapefruit essential oil

5 drops Bergamot essential oil

Instructions

1. Mix the oils together and use several drops in an inhaler.

Alertness And Energizing Blend

Faced with a demanding task? Use this blend when and you will be w mentally alert and aware.

14 drops Juniper essential oil

8 drops Rosemary essential oil

8 drops Pine needle essential oil

Instructions

1. Blend all the ingredients in a dark bottle.

2. Place several drops in your home, office or car diffuser (for long distance driving).

3. When diffusing in the car, use only for 20 minutes at a time.

Concentration Enhancing Blend

20 drops Lemon essential oil

6 drops Basil essential oil

2 drops Rosemary essential oil

Instructions

1. Mix these essential oils together then diffuse into the air.

2. If you are at work, you can place a personal diffuser on your desk or just put a few drops of the blend on tissue for inhaling.

Anxiety Relief Recipe

It is not always possible to avoid things that make you anxious. You can however handle uncertainties better when you use nerve-calming essential oils.

2 drops Geranium essential oil

2 drops Vanilla essential oil

3 drops Neroli essential oil

2 drops Rosewood essential oil

1 drops Frankincense essential oil

2 drops Ylang ylang essential oil

1 drop Rose essential oil

Instructions

1. Mix properly in dark glass bottle.

2. Use in a nasal inhaler or just place 1-2 drops on tissue or cotton ball and inhale.

Aromatherapy For Burnout, Exhaustion And Fatigue

These oils can rejuvenate and lift you up when you have been through a physically and mentally exhaustive circumstance.

15 drops Lime essential oil

8 drops Grapefruit essential oil

8 drops Cardamom essential oil

Instructions

1. Add a few drops into a diffuser in the room where you are resting.

2. Mix with 2 ounces of almond oil and treat yourself to a relaxing massage to release tense muscles.

Note: Exhaustion and burnout will require several days of adequate rest and sleep.

Romantic Massage Blend

Several essential oils can enhance the feeling of excitement and stimulate sensations for romantic encounters.

2 drops Orange essential oil

2 drops Jasmine essential oil

1 drop Ylang ylang essential oil

2 drops Sandalwood essential oil

1 ounce Almond oil -

Instructions

1. Mix the ingredients properly.

2. Use for a slow and loving, romantic massage.

Memory Loss Recovery Blend

Memory loss is predominant in the elderly but it can also be experienced occasionally by younger people. Essential oils like Rosemary and Basil are used for dementia and Alzheimer's patients in many nursing facilities.

6 drops Basil essential oil -

20 drops Lemon essential oil

2 drops Rosemary essential oil

Instructions

1. Mix the oils together and use in a diffuser.

Aphrodisiac For Love And Romance

3 drops Sandalwood essential oil

2 drops Rose essential oil

1 or 2 tablespoons Lotion

Instructions

1. Mix the essential oils into 1 or 2 tablespoons of your body lotion.

2. Apply on your arms, face and body.

Panic And Panic Attacks Bath Oil

12 drops Lavender essential oil

3 drops Rose essential oil

2 ounces Jojoba oil

Instructions

1. Mix essential oils with Jojoba in a dark glass bottle.

2. Add 1-2 teaspoons to your bath water.

Panic And Panic Attacks Diffuser Blend

Use this blend in times of panic.

16 drops Lavender essential oil

4 drops Rose essential oil

Instructions

1. Add oils to a dark glass bottle and shake together.

2. Use this blend in your diffuser.

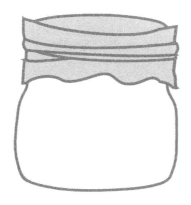

Seasonal Affective Disorder (SAD) And Cabin Fever

It is natural for some people to have the blues for one or two days when the seasons are changing.

15 drops Geranium essential oil

10 drops Bergamot essential oil

5 drops Lavender essential oil -

Instructions

1. Blend the oils together and use in a diffuser.

2. Add 6-8 drops of this blend to the bath tub and soak in the water.

Note: Endeavor to go outside within the daylight hours to make you feel better during this time.

Confidence Boosting Rub

20 drops Rosemary essential oil

10 drops Fennel essential oil

2 ounces Carrier oil or lotion -

Instructions

1. Mix together the ingredients and apply to your skin when needed.

Happiness Enhancing Blend

Although essential oils cannot create happiness, they can help to clear your mind so you can focus on things that make you happy. Use the following blend to bring up your spirits.

5 drops Rose geranium essential oil

19 drops Orange essential oil

1 drop Cinnamon essential oil

1 drop Clove essential oil

Instructions

1. Blend these oils and use in a diffuser.

2. Use 5 drops in your bath.

Positive Energy Recipe

4 drops Orange essential oil

3 drops Lavender essential oil

1or 2 drops Rose essential oil

Instructions

1. Add these essential oils to 2 ounces of distilled water in a spray bottle.

2. Spray often in your work area.

Overcoming Insecurity

Essential oils can help to enhance self confidence and strengthen your emotions when you are feeling insecure.

2 drops Bergamot essential oil

2 drops Cedarwood essential oil

1 drop Frankincense essential oil

Instructions

1. Multiply this recipe by 4 to make 20 drops. Keep in a dark glass bottle then use the necessary number of drops in a diffuser.

2. For bath oil, multiply this recipe by 3 to make 15 drops then mix with 2 ounces of Jojoba oil in a dark glass bottle. Use 1-2 teaspoonfuls per bath.

Comfort For Grief And Loss

It is natural to go through a period of grief when you lose a loved one, a job or a pet. Essential oils can help with the sorrow and sadness being experienced at this time.

5 drops Vanilla essential oil

3 drops Mandarin essential oil

3 drops Rose Otto essential oil

3 drops Roman Chamomile essential oil

Instructions

1. Blend the oils in a dark glass bottle and use in your diffuser.

2. Blend oils with 1 ounce of Almond or Jojoba oil and use for massage.

Insomnia Massage Blend

1 drop Marjoram essential oil

1 drop Ylang Ylang essential oil

1 drop Roman Chamomile essential oil

1 drop Sweet Orange essential oil

1 drop Tangerine essential oil

1 drop Lavender essential oil

1 ounce Carrier oil

Instructions

1. Mix the oils together and massage your body at bedtime.

Insomnia Sleep Time Blend

Avoid stimulating foods like coffee, colas and some evening teas when you use this blend. Additionally, avoid stimulating entertainment (movies or talk shows) close to bedtime.

6 drops Sandalwood essential oil

2 drops Ylang Ylang essential oil

2 drops Neroli essential oil

1 drop Vetiver essential oil

1 drop Coriander essential oil

1 tablespoon Jojoba oil -

Instructions

1. Blend essential oils with Jojoba.

2. Take a warm bath before bedtime then apply this blend to pulse points such as inside of the wrists, behind the ears and behind the knees.

Nervousness And Anxiety

10 drops Lavender essential oil

10 drops Orange essential oil

2 drops Marjoram essential oil

2 drops Cedarwood essential oil

4 ounces Sweet Almond oil

Instructions

1. Combine ingredients in a small glass bottle.

2. Open and inhale whenever you feel nervous.

Loneliness Diffuser Blend

8 drops Bergamot essential oil

8 drops Frankincense essential oil

4drops Rose essential oil

Instructions

1. Mix together properly in a dark bottle.

2. Use appropriate drops in a diffuser.

Jetlag

Jetlag occurs when your body's psychological and physiological rhythms are disrupted due to long flights taken. The symptoms include sleep disturbance, fatigue, aching or swollen feet and nausea.

Instructions

1. During the flight, massage your feet with 1 drop of Geranium, Grapefruit or Basil oil diluted with a dash of carrier oil.

2. On arrival, put 10 drops of Lavender oil in your hand and rub on the torso to stay alert and then shower immediately.

3. Revive your mind and body by adding the oils below to a warm bath. Enjoy

2 drops Peppermint essential oil

1 drop Bergamot essential oil

1 drop Rosemary essential oil

1 drop Geranium essential oil

2 drops Neroli essential oil

Stress Eliminating Recipe

15 drops Lavender essential oil

10 drops Lemon essential oil

5 drops Clary Sage essential oil

Instructions

1. Mix together in an amber bottle.

2. Use in a diffuser or personal nasal inhaler.

3. Add 5-6 drops of this blend to warm bath water and soak in it for 20-30 minutes.

Loneliness Bath Oil

6 drops Bergamot essential oil

6 drops Frankincense essential oil

3 drop Rose essential oil

2 ounces Jojoba oil

Instructions

1. Blend oils together in a dark glass bottle.

2. Use 1-2 teaspoonfuls in your bath water.

Concentration Spray

Fight after-lunch sleepiness with this remedy

2 drops Peppermint

3 drops Lemon

3 drops Rosemary

2 cups water

Instructions

1. Add the oils to water and spray around your office or home.

Emotional Shock Relief

Emotional shock can occur when you hear bad news or experience a negative occurrence. The following essential oils can help you to calm down until normalcy returns.

Lavender

Neroli

Tea Tree

Rose

Roman Chamomile

Instructions

1. Keep a vial of any of these oils in a purse or pocket.

2. Place a few drops on tissue or cotton ball and inhale. You could also use a nasal inhaler.

3. Mix any of the oils with a little carrier oil for a back rub or foot rub.

Release Sexual Energy

2 drop of Sandalwood

2 drops Rosemary

2 drops Jasmine

2 teaspoons jojoba oil

Instructions

Combine the essential oils in a simmer pot or diffuser.

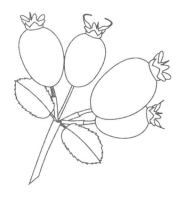

Painful Periods/Cramps

2-4 drops Clary Sage/Cypress

Instructions

1. Apply topically to the abdomen.

2. Next, use a warm compress on the abdomen.

Menstrual Cramps Bath Remedy

5 drops Lavender

2 drops Cypress

2 drops Nutmeg

2 drops Peppermint

1/2 cup Epsom and/or sea salt

Instructions:

1. Combine oils and add to bath salts.

2. Soak for 20- 30 min. Rinse and take a rest, elevating your legs

Vaginitis (Virginal Inflammation)

75% of women will experience this condition in their lifetime. it is mostly caused by a bacteria and very rarely fungal infection.

2 - 5 drops Lavender

2 - 5 drops Melaleuca

1 tablespoon (1/2 ounce) Extra Virgin Coconut Oil

Instructions

1. Add essential oils to coconut oil. Soak into a tampon.

2. Use nightly for a week

Varicose Veins Essential Oil Blend

Veins in the body may become weakened with time and lots of pressure. As a result, they become enlarged and twisted.

30 drops Cypress essential oil

20 drops Lavender

10 drops Lemon essential oil

2 oz Coconut oil

Instructions

1. Blend all and apply morning and night. Improvement will be noticeable in about a month.

2. When this happens, apply daily for 3 or 4 months more.

Mood Soother For PMS

PMS is the acronym for premenstrual syndrome. It comprises various symptoms that generally begin several days before menstruation. These symptoms include breast swelling and tenderness, water retention, depression, irritability, headaches and mood swings.

9 drops Geranium essential oil

6 drops Chamomile essential oil

3 drops Clary sage essential oil

3 drops Angelica essential oil (if available)

2 drops Marjoram essential oil

2 ounces Vegetable essential oil

Instructions

1. Combine all ingredients. The angelica oil works real well but it is optional because it may be hard to find.

2. Add 1- 2 teaspoons to bath or use as massage oil. For more effectiveness, add 1- 2 drops of neroli, jasmine or rose. Without the vegetable oil, it can be used in a diffuser or place in a vial to smell as needed.

Vaginal Candida Or Yeast Infection Douche

1 drop Geranium essential oil

2 drops Tea Tree essential oil

2 drops Rosemary essential oil

2 drops Lavender essential oil

2 tablespoons Vinegar

3 cups Lukewarm water

Instructions

1. Mix ingredients together.

2. Use once daily as a douche or Sitz bath.

Candida Or Yeast Infection

5 drops Lemon essential oil

5 drops Melaleuca essential oil

3 drops Oregano essential oil

Instructions

1. Add the essential oils to a gel cap then take internally two times daily for about 10 to 14 days.

2. Take a two weeks break then repeat the procedure.

The End

Made in the USA
Monee, IL
29 May 2023